GETTING YOUNGER IS NOT A DREAM

WHAT YOU SHOULD KNOW ABOUT GETTING OLDER, HOW YOU CAN PREVENT IT AND HOW YOU CAN EVEN GET YOUNGER AGAIN. / THE »FOUNTAIN OF YOUTH - PROGRAM«

PETER CARL SIMONS

Copyright © Peter Carl Simons
All Rights Reserved.

ISBN 978-1-63920-302-4

This book has been published with all efforts taken to make the material error-free after the consent of the author. However, the author and the publisher do not assume and hereby disclaim any liability to any party for any loss, damage, or disruption caused by errors or omissions, whether such errors or omissions result from negligence, accident, or any other cause.

While every effort has been made to avoid any mistake or omission, this publication is being sold on the condition and understanding that neither the author nor the publishers or printers would be liable in any manner to any person by reason of any mistake or omission in this publication or for any action taken or omitted to be taken or advice rendered or accepted on the basis of this work. For any defect in printing or binding the publishers will be liable only to replace the defective copy by another copy of this work then available.

Contents

FOREWORD

Good morning, dear readers,

Everyone wants to get old - nobody wants to be old. That is how the folk saying goes and, in fact, this is so because »being old« in our experience is about frailty, disease, limited mobility, dementia and short life expectancy.

When I came across an article on the discovery of the Nobel laureates Elizabeth H. Blackburn, Jack W. Szostak, and Carol W. Greidler two years ago, my interest was piqued. The three researchers received the Nobel prize for medicine in 2009. Their research was on "how chromosomes are protected by telomeres and the enzyme telomerase". What sounds incomprehensible, is an important step towards the discovery of the »fountain of youth«, as I will explain later.

In research there are, in fact, two fundamental theories_[1], that describe why the human body becomes frailer as it is getting older and eventually dies. One is the damage theory, which assumes that the body is especially destroyed by free radicals over time, and the other one is the telomere hypothesis, according to which errors creep into the ongoing renewal of cells over time, whereby the body suffers from more and more micro-defects and eventually reaches a fatal damage.

The »fountain of youth - program«_[2] that I developed, takes the findings of both theories and works with targeted measures against aging, which will also help you to reach an old age full of health and activity - even if the latter is currently not the case. This is, thus, not about prevention, but successes of users show that even already existing damages can be repaired to a large extent.

I hope that I have piqued your interest and am glad if the following pages help you to considerably increase your health up until old age. Of course, the book cannot replace advice from an expert. Therefore, I have deliberately refrained from mentioning certain products or amounts. Agree upon those with an expert of your choice.

I wish you a lot of success with that.

Yours, Peter Carl Simons

[1]In fact, there is a variety of further theories, which can, however, in their essence be reduced to the formerly mentioned. Many others only enjoy little acceptance in the world of research.

[2]I have called it that because everyone understands what it means.

I

What does »aging« mean?

As long as there are people who are aware that they age and eventually will die one day, some search for the fountain of youth with which they are able to prevent or at least delay aging. World history is full of people that invest time, money and a lot of energy in order to »live forever«.

But what does aging actually mean? Regarding that Wikipedia writes:

Ageing (British English) or aging (American English) is the process of becoming older. In the narrow sense, the term refers to biological ageing of human beings, animals and other organisms. In the broader sense, ageing can refer to single cells within an organism (cellular ageing) or to the population of a species (population ageing).

In humans, ageing represents the accumulation of changes in a human being over time, encompassing physical, psychological, and social change. Reaction time, for example, may slow with age, while knowledge of world events and wisdom may expand. Ageing is among the greatest known risk factors for most human diseases: of the roughly 150,000 people who die each day across the globe, about two thirds die from age-related causes.

The causes of ageing are unknown; current theories are assigned to the damage concept, whereby the accumulation of externally induced damage (such as DNA point mutations) may cause biological systems to fail, or to the programmed ageing concept, whereby internal processes (such as DNA telomere shortening) may cause ageing.

Therefore, aging is basically about the body being damaged in the context of changes over the course of time. These damages are the reason for why it does not function optimally anymore and in turn, further damages occur. This goes on until a system-relevant organ (e.g. the brain) or the entire system is so damaged that the body is not capable of continuing to work and »shuts down«.

Since 1970, the average life expectancy of humans has increased by about ten years in most Western European countries. At the same time, the statistics, however, show that also the time of people being ill or injured has increased.[1]

What many people do not know is the fact that »aging« and »dying« does not affect all living things on this planet. Single-celled organisms, algae or freshwater polyps do not age. The physical decay is a process that seems to be reserved for creatures that reproduce through sexual reproduction. This finding has led to two basic theories that are supposed to explain aging and the aging process.

[1]See »World Health Report« of the WHO – can be downloaded on http://www.who.int/ for free.

II

The damage theory

The damage theory can be easily explained based on an image. Imagine you park your beautiful, freshly washed car openly in the desert. With every sandstorm, millions of small stone pieces patter on the paint. The first thousand might do no damage, but over time, the paint will get a little damaged. Finally, the paint becomes matt and even chips after some time. Your car is probably still roadworthy (or it only needs new tires). But if the car is parked in the desert any longer, the sand will over time erode the metal and over millions and millions of micro-impacts even remove it until the car (in extreme cases) is completely destroyed. Even the biggest sandstorm will not achieve that over night, but perhaps over the course of 50 or 100 years?

The damage theory basically says the same. But with our body, it is not about sand, but about substances that damage or impair our cells. The most common damage theory is the theory of »free radicals«. This came up during the mid-20th century.

Free radicals, therefore, damage various molecules - including the nucleic acid which forms our genetic information within the DNA. As with the example of the sand grains, the first free radical does not lead to lasting damage. But »constant dripping wears the stone« applies here. Over time, cells, cell aggregates or entire organs can be damaged so much, that they lose their function.

The damage theory is used as an explanation of various diseases, such as cancer, diabetes or Alzheimer's.

The body, however, is able to reduce the negative effects of free radicals. For this, it needs the necessary nutrients. These are called antioxidants and are described on Wikipedia as follows:

An antioxidant is a molecule that inhibits the oxidation of other molecules. Oxidation is a chemical reaction that can produce free radicals, leading to chain reactions that may damage cells. Antioxidants such as thiols or ascorbic acid (vitamin C) terminate these chain reactions.

To balance the oxidative state, plants and animals maintain complex systems of overlapping antioxidants, such as glutathione and enzymes (e.g., catalase and superoxide dismutase) produced internally or vitamin C, vitamin A and vitamin E obtained by ingestion.

Diets containing foods high in antioxidants have been shown to improve health. However, in supplement form, the prevention of diseases such as cancer or coronary heart disease and the general promotion of health has not been confirmed experimentally. Trials including supplements of beta-carotene, vitamin A, and vitamin E singly or in different combinations found no effect on mortality or might increase it. Randomized clinical trials of taking antioxidants including beta-carotene, vitamin E, vitamin C and selenium have shown no effect on cancer risk or have increased cancer risk. Supplementation with selenium or vitamin E does not reduce the risk of cardiovascular disease. Oxidative stress can be considered as either a cause or consequence of some diseases, stimulating drug development for potential antioxidant compounds for use as treatments.

III

The telomere hypothesis

The telomere hypothesis and the damage theory complement each other perfectly. It is not that only one or the other might be right. The telomere hypothesis goes back to the American gerontologist Leonard Hayflick, who already recognized in 1961 that cells cannot divide indefinitely. This phenomenon can also be illustrated by an image.

When you photocopy a document and make a copy of the resulting photocopy - and, thus, create hundreds or thousands of photocopies -, you will soon notice that even with the best photocopier (or scanner and printer) it will come to quality losses. Even if a copy displayed 99,9 percent of the original, the quality would decrease over time until a clear difference can even be seen with the naked eye.

With his research, Hayflick found out that cells can divide themselves up to 50 times. Assuming that the human body consists of about 100 trillion cells (that are 100 000 000 000 000 cells), it does not seem particularly threatening when a cell is defective after 50 divisions. But since our body performs 10 million cell divisions per second, one can imagine that this effect may become a problem after some time.

The telomere hypothesis was confirmed in 1991 by the later Nobel laureate in medicine, Jack William Szostak, with research findings. In an article, that was published in that year, he showed how telomeres constantly shorten in the cell.

Telomeres and telomerase

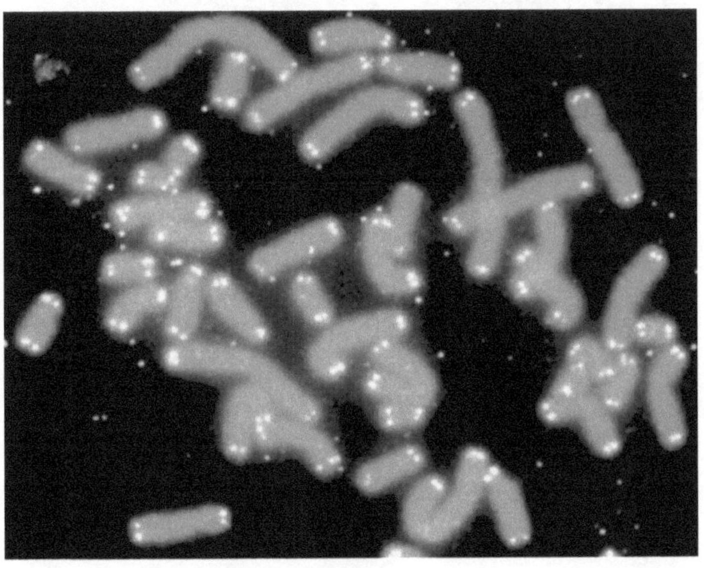

But what are telomeres and telomerase and what does all this have to do with aging? In order to understand that, we have to deal with the structure and function of our cells.

Within every human cell is a program that establishes how the cell looks and how it behaves. This program is called DNA, which stands for deoxyribonucleic acid. The DNA is in the nucleus. Its molecular structure has already been deciphered in 1953 by James D. Watson and Francis Crick.

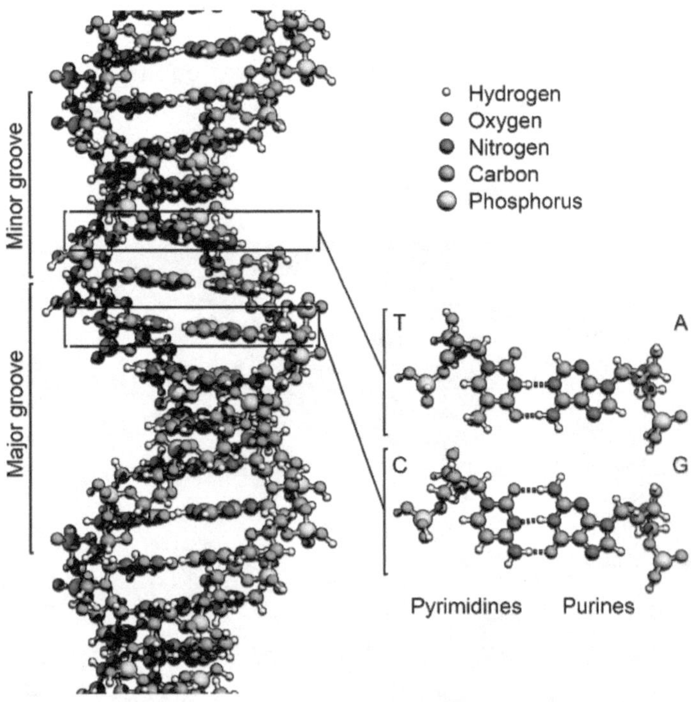

The DNA forms a double-strand which looks like a twisted ladder. Its steps consist of four different types of molecules. Here, the respective molecules of both strands complement each other and form pairs.

For cell division, the strands group into the X-shaped chromosomes, with which the telomeres form the outer ends. They form a kind of protective cap that ensures that the chromosomes do not inadvertently connect with others which lead to changes in the genetic information. Already in the 70s, the researchers Watson and Olonikov showed that with every cell division a small piece of the chromosomes is not copied (remember the photocopier element).

This part, which is not copied, is part of the telomeres. If these are »depleted«, the actual genetic information is damaged during the copying process (which is the basis of human life) and corresponding damages follow. The enzyme telomerase can, however, restore the full length of the telomeres and, thus, prevent the degradation of the cell. It was identified in 1991 and is only formed in certain cells, for example in immune cells or embryonic stem cells.

research has shown that shortened telomeres highly correlate with various diseases. These include cancer tumors as well as organ defects or circulatory disorders. Short: The majority of results confirm the telomere hypothesis. If a certain number of cell divisions was carried out, it leads to a damage of the chromosomes and, thus, to malfunction, aging and ultimately to death.

By now, it is hardly known that also plant substances can reverse the damage to the telomeres. The following chapters are going to be about these.

IV
Astragalus membranaceus, Astragalus

The Astragalus root, scientifically called Astragalus membranaceus, is colloquially also known as Astragalus. It has its origins in Eastern Chine, where it was given the translated name »yellow sacred old boy«. Chinese folk medicine and traditional Chinese medicine (TCM) have been using it in various areas for a long time. Usually, the root is used.

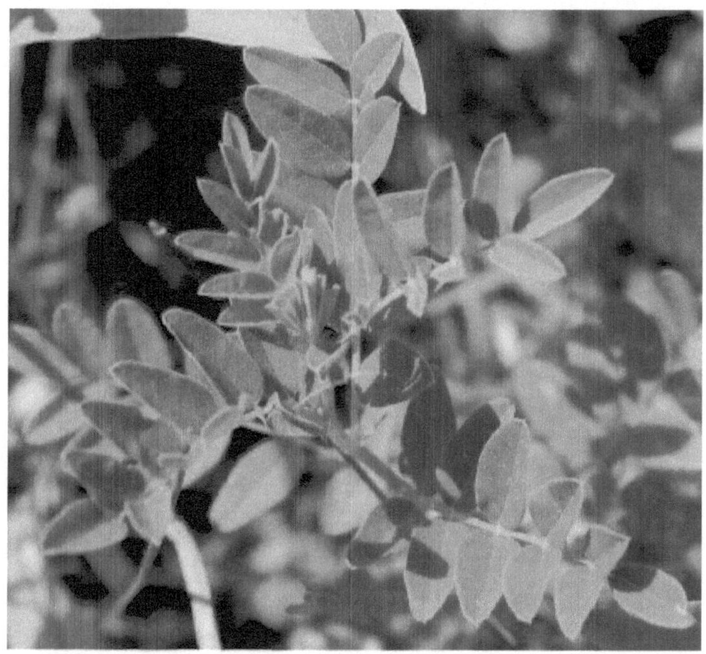

The most important components of the root are flavonoids, saponins, polysaccharides, amino acids, mineral substances, trace elements, and vitamins. It can be used respectively versatile. It is not surprising that in Asia several mixtures against a SARS infection contained this versatile root.

In summary, it can be said that the ingredients of the Astragalus root have among others the following benefits:

- antiviral effect
- antioxidant (field of topic: »free radicals«)
- antitumor-forming (prevents or reduces the formation of tumors)

- anti-inflammatory
- increase in formation of telomerase (field of topic: »telomere depletion«)

V

Which effects has the Astragalus root?

Like many natural products, the root of the Astragalus membranaceus plant contains a variety of active ingredients. Based on the knowledge of the traditional Chinese medicine and on the scientific research from the rest of the world, the following five effects can be seen, which the following sections will explain further.

Antiviral effect

Research has proven a positive influence of the Astragalus root on various viral diseases. It helps to combat the HIV virus, hepatitis B, and viral myocardial inflammation.

Antioxidant effect – fighting the free radicals

Astragalus has a strong antioxidant effect. The contained polysaccharides are used to protect the mitochondria of the cell, which slows down the aging process.

Antitumor effect

Malignant tumors commonly referred to as cancer, mean a considerable health impairment. More and more sufferers want to be treated with medication.

Currently, it is intensively researched how the Astragalus root can be used for treating tumors. There are already results for supplementing conventional therapies with the active agents of the root. The researched cases, the side effects of the conventional therapy decreased, which considerably improved the quality of life of the patients.

Anti-inflammatory effect

Inflammations are immune reactions of the body. They can be caused by many different reasons and can be the reaction to injuries, poisoning or pathogens. The local inflammation is supposed to kill impurities and repair the body. Fever is, therefore, also an inflammation, which, however, affects the whole body because the pathogen is not only present locally (as with an injury), but attack many parts of the body.

While a short-term inflammation can be helpful and belongs to the healthy functioning of the body, chronic inflammations are not useful. These can be caused by various factors. One is self-poisoning based on intestinal problems (see chapter 7, step 1: bowel repair). Another increasingly widespread inflammation is a chronic inflammation of considerably overweight people. There, the immune cells are often permanently activated. Renowned researchers consider this the reason for why diabetes is developed.

The active ingredients contained in the Astragalus root, on the one hand, reduce blood sugar and blood lipid levels, which reduces the risk of diabetes. And on the other hand, they have an anti-inflammatory effect. Especially less pro-inflammatory proteins are produced in the intestinal cells.

Increase in telomerase formation

If we want to counteract the aging process of our cells in order to reach positive influences on our life expectancy and health, an increased formation of telomerase is of particular importance.

Telomerase can not only protect the telomeres (i.e. the ends of the chromosomes) during cell division but also repair them. Thus, experiments on organs have proven that substances of the Astragalus root have a rejuvenating effect.

To put it plainly: So far, there is no evidence for the claim that people could live longer because of the consumption of the Astragalus root or its extracts. That is impossible because it cannot be tested how »the same person« leads a live with and a live without the substances.

Seen this way, every application of the Astragalus root is speculative in terms of life extension. Numerous applications of users show, however, that many people, who regularly consumed high-quality Astragalus extract were more powerful and that they significantly reduced their biological age.

Especially athletes use the »fountain of youth - program« in order to keep their body fit for a longer time. Of course, this is not considered doping.

Finally, it remains up to you, whether you want to use Astragalus membranaceus or not. No one can guarantee a specific success. But many positive experiences increase the probability.

VI

The »fountain of youth - program«

Countless people still have a very mechanistic self-image: If the foot hurts, they cure the foot; if they have a headache, they take headache pills; and if they do not want to age prematurely, they resort to anti-aging preparations twice a day.

In many cases these people find that their therapy is not sustainable: The headache is gone for today, but after a few days or weeks it comes back; the foot stops hurting for a short time, but swells uncomfortably and the anti-aging also does not seem to work. No wonder: If we want to only begin to understand our body and its diseases, we have to look at it as an entire system.

It may be that someone has back pain because his knee is injured. Then that leg is, thus, less strained and all back muscles are tensed. Of course, you can now massage the back and rub it with ointment, perhaps even take some medication, but you still follow the wrong goal. Only when the knee is healthy and the body has also »understood« that, the legs will go normal again and the reason for the back pain is gone (assuming that there is no second reason).

Another example are headaches. In fact, it often happens that headaches are the result of bowel problems. This might sound odd, but it is reality. The intestine is a wonderful system and Julia Enders has drawn a wonderful »portrait« of this organ with her book »Gut: The Inside Story of Our Body's Most Underrated Organ«, which has been on the Spiegel bestseller list for months.

However, the intestine cannot optimally function if there are fungal infections, rotting herds, oproliths and silting in it. Especially rotting herds in the intestine can lead to a gradual self-poisoning of the body. The rotting substances are absorbed by the intestine just as good nutrients are and travel through the bloodstream into all body parts - in some cases even into the head where they can cause a headache. These toxins can also cause pain, inflammations and many diseases up to cancer in other body regions.

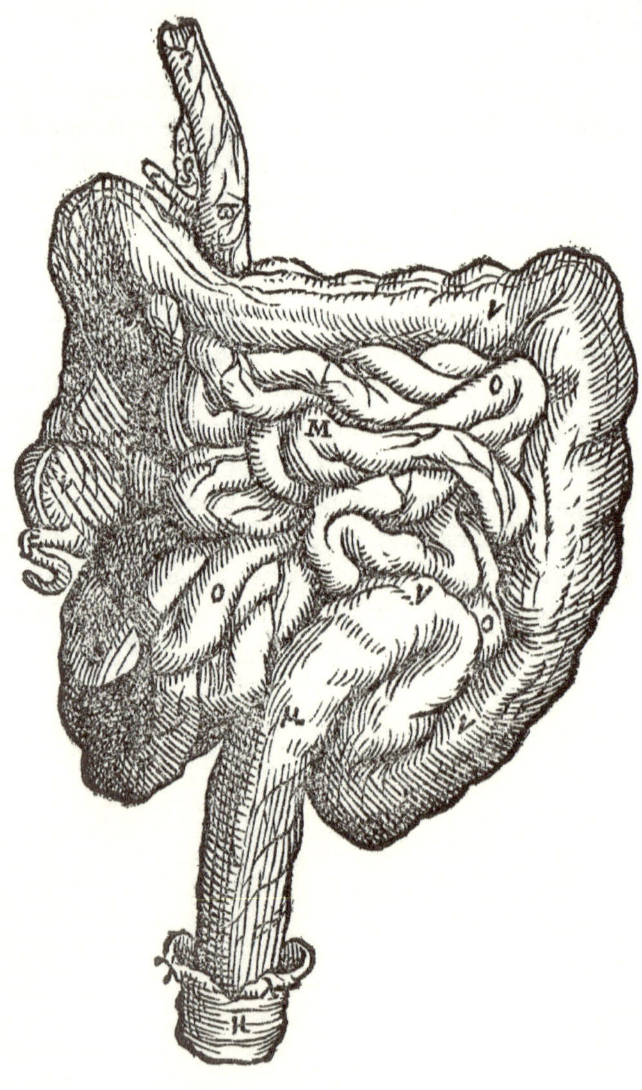

It, therefore, is not enough to work on your telomeres being »of excellent health« if you poison them at the same time. For that reason, intestinal repair is always the first step of the »fountain of youth - program«.

Step 1: Intestinal repair

A successful repair of the intestine is based on three elements:

- dietary fiber for the stimulation of the bowel function
- secondary plant compounds for detoxification
- substances for a deacidification because with overacidification the intestinal villi are attacked and lastingly damaged

A separate book will be devoted to this topic, which will explain all relations in detail. That is why I will only look at the main aspects in this guide._[1]

Generally, it is recommended to cleanse one's intestine once a year during one month.

Dietary fiber

Fiber plays an important role for the intestine. A healthy colon has to stay in movement. For that, the mentioned substances are designated. Of these, we consume fewer and fewer in our modern society.

Wikipedia on dietary fiber:

Dietary fiber or roughage is the indigestible portion of food derived from plants. It has two main components:

Soluble fiber, which dissolves in water, is readily fermented in the colon into gases and physiologically active byproducts, and can be prebiotic and viscous.

Insoluble fiber, which does not dissolve in water, is metabolically inert and provides bulking, or it can be prebiotic and metabolically ferment in the large intestine. Bulking fibers absorb water as they move through the digestive system, easing defecation.

Dietary fibers can act by changing the nature of the contents of the gastrointestinal tract and by changing how other nutrients and chemicals are absorbed. Some types of soluble fiber absorb water to become a gelatinous, viscous substance which is fermented by bacteria in the digestive tract. Some types of insoluble fiber have bulking action and are not fermented. Lignin, a major dietary insoluble fiber source, may alter the rate and metabolism of soluble fibers.[Other types of insoluble fiber, notably resistant starch, are fully fermented. Some but not all soluble plant fibers block intestinal mucosal adherence and translocation of potentially pathogenic bacteria and may therefore modulate intestinal inflammation, an effect that has been termed contrabiotic.

Chemically, dietary fiber consists of non-starch polysaccharides such as arabinoxylans, cellulose, and many other plant components such as resistant starch, resistant dextrins, inulin, lignin, chitins, pectins, beta-glucans, and oligosaccharides. A novel position has been adopted by the US Department of Agriculture to include functional fibers as isolated fiber sources that may be included in the diet. The term "fiber" is something of a misnomer, since many types of so-called dietary fiber are not actually fibrous.

Food sources of dietary fiber are often divided according to whether they provide (predominantly) soluble or insoluble fiber. Plant foods contain both types of fiber in varying degrees, according to the plant's characteristics.

Advantages of consuming fiber are the production of healthful compounds during the fermentation of soluble fiber, and insoluble fiber's ability (via its passive hygroscopic properties) to increase bulk, soften stool, and shorten transit time through the intestinal tract. A disadvantage of a diet high in fiber is the potential for significant intestinal gas production and bloating.

Dietary fiber should ideally be ingested through a healthy diet. An assortment of products and their fiber can also be found on Wikipedia:

Food group	Serving Mean	fiber g/serving
Fruit	0.5 cup	1.1
Dark-green vegetables	0.5 cup	6.4
Orange vegetables	0.5 cup	2.1
Cooked dry beans (legumes)	0.5 cup	8.0

Food group	Serving Mean	fiber g/serving
Starchy vegetables	0.5 cup	1.7
Other vegetables	0.5 cup	1.1
Whole grains	28 g (1 oz)	2.4
Meat	28 g (1 oz)	0.1

In fact, only very few people constantly consume enough fiber. The daily tablespoon wheat bran does neither harmoniously blend in with our diet, nor is this one-sided supply of fiber optimal. Ideally, it is a mixture of different fibers. Some well-known suppliers have developed appropriate products which often also comprise a basic supply of vital substances.

Detoxification

In the context of a repairing the intestine, the detoxification occupies a special place. Many people carry a lot of bacteria, fungi, and parasites in their intestine, which do not belong there and which can sustainably damage the body.

Adverse residents include putrefactive bacteria, whose growth is mainly promoted by an excessive consumption of meat and dairy products. In fact, there no or only little putrefaction in a healthy intestine. This has various effects.

The most obvious effect is the odor development. In severe cases, it goes as far that the body emits these odors even with the sweat. With that, even the biggest cloud of perfume only helps temporarily. But much more dangerous is that with the putrefaction substances develop that are absorbed by the blood and, thus, they are transported into the entire body. there, they can lead to various secondary diseases.

Fungal infections in the intestine are mainly the result of an excessive consumption of carbohydrates, especially of baked goods. These provide the optimal nutrition for the fungi which grow rampantly in our intestine and not only prevent the intestine from doing its normal »work«, but also provide an ideal home for other substances and parasites. They can cause self-poisoning as well.

A third problem is parasites. Most people only know of the tapeworm, although it is a whole family of more than 3000 species.

These fellows, which are partly »unpleasant« and sometimes even harmful to health, are, in fact, only a small part of the parasites which can colonize the intestine. For some, the human intestine is only an intermediate host. Others, on the other hand, drill through the intestinal wall or lead to other considerable damages. Various plant products and mixtures counteract that well and in many cases make chemical treatment unnecessary.

Deacidification

Deacidification and other therapies, based on dietary fiber and the detoxification of the body, are often inexplicably treated separately. Many providers of programs make this mistake.

One author, who consistently brings both topics together, is Frank Schmidt with his book on HCG-colon repair._[2] The approach described there is convincing and coincides for most parts with my ideas, although the intake of »HCG« is seen there in the context of weight reduction. If you want to repair your intestine in order to lose weight, I recommend the book by Frank Schmidt to you.

There are undoubtedly many products and whole product families for deacidification. All of them (which are useful) are based on the knowledge that we consume highly acidic foods in our society today. It is fact that because of environmental pollution and the resulting acid rain our foods are significantly more sour than they were a few centuries ago. Dietary changes as for example the high consumption of carbonated drinks support the daily acidic attack even more.

One can counteract this overacidification in different ways and there are different natural products available on the market.

Step 2: providing a base of vital substances

Imagine you want to build a house and have all construction material on site. Only the deliverer, who delivers your mortar, does not come. Now, you could start to pile the bricks and put the mortar in between later on. But experience teaches us that a solid house is not built this way.

It is similar in our body. Within it, billions of processes take place every second and many of them need certain bricks. Whether cells divide, dead cells are disposed or cells are supplied with nutrients - in order for the processes to function well, vital substances are necessary. If a substance is missing, the body will slow down this process or not conduct it at all. The consequences can be diseases, lack of energy or the like.

Anyone who deals with the literature and the results of research on the topic of vital substances quickly realizes that certain daily doses are recommended. Some research findings also suggest that an increased intake of certain substances offers considerable advantages.

Basically, it makes sense to ensure that the recommended daily allowance of the different vital substances, such as vitamins, trace elements, mineral substances, etc. is available for the body. In addition, there is plenty of very good literature on vital substances, which I want to entrust to you.

In the context of the fountain of youth program, it is usually worked with a broadband vital substance preparation in combination with OPC and MSM. For that, talk to your nutritionist or physician, depending on where you feel more comfortable.

Step 3: The Astragalus cure

In order for your body to efficiently use Astragalus, you need to provide it with sufficient nutrients. Only with the help of vital substances our body is capable of using the other substances optimally. This also applies to the active ingredients of the Astragalus root. Thus, it is recommended to ensure a sufficient supply of vital substances.

Instead of buying entire Astragalus roots, it is advisable to use a high-quality Astragalus extract. In the extract, the active ingredients are optimally concentrated. High-quality products are partly offered for enormous prices of far more than 10,000 euros per monthly dose. Fortunately, there are also high-quality offers in a range that are affordable for average earners. For more information, look at the reference sources.

In the context of the fountain of youth program a preparation with Astragalus root and further valuable substances is used, which combination has particularly positive results.

[1]The serves the purpose of better readability in order to create a rather comprehensible and uncomplicated guide. A intestinal repair is very useful and recommended also in other contexts than the »fountain of youth program«.

[2]Schmidt, Frank: Die HCG-Darmreinigung: Ihre Grundlage für doppelten Erfolg in der Stoffwechselkur. – Warum eine Stoffwechselkur nach fachlicher Darmreinigung viel erfolgreicher ist., BOD, 2015.

www.ingramcontent.com/pod-product-compliance
Lightning Source LLC
Chambersburg PA
CBHW051405250726
48656CB00006B/2280